Beyond Cannabis

Halt Autoimmune, Metabolic and Neurodegenerative Disease with Common Terpenes, Polyphenols and Dietary Cannabinoids

Anne Angelone

Copyright © by Anne Angelone 2016

All Rights Reserved

ISBN-13: 978-1535253376
ISBN-10: 1535253371

Disclaimer: This guide is not intended to provide medical advice or to take the place of medical advice and treatment from your personal physician. Readers are advised to consult their own doctors or other qualified health professionals regarding the treatment of medical conditions.

The author shall not be held liable or responsible for any misunderstanding or misuse of the information contained in this manual or for any loss, damage, or injury caused or alleged to be caused directly or indirectly by any treatment, action, or application of any food or food source discussed in this program manual. The information in this guide has not been evaluated by the U.S. Food and Drug Administration. This information is not intended to diagnose, treat, cure, or prevent any disease.

To request permission for reproduction, please contact:
Website: www.beyondcannabis.club

CONTENTS

The discovery that different plants beyond cannabis contain multiple compounds that can modulate the endocannabinoid system means that we can no longer define plant cannabinoids as merely a product of cannabis

~Juerg Gertsch

INTRODUCTION

As research into medical cannabis continues to capture the attention of many in the scientific and medical communities (as well as many in the general public), we are also learning more about the health benefits brought on by the best combination of non-cannabis botanical compounds, foods, and lifestyle activities (e.g., acupuncture, exercise, and aromatherapy) that interact with the endocannabinoid system (ECS).

The ECS is a lipid-signaling network that regulates most metabolic, immune, neurodegenerative and inflammatory diseases. You can think of it as the global system in our body that naturally produces ligands (binding molecules) that activate the receptors that regulates inflammatory cytokines, lipid, and sugar and neurotransmitter release. And, because the ECS is responsible for neural plasticity, neuroprotection, immunity and inflammation, apoptosis, pain, appetite, and metabolism (McPartland, 2008), supporting this system is important for halting chronic disease expression.

Although we have *Cannabis sativa* to thank for much of the emerging information about and interest in the ECS, we are now discovering that plants and compounds other than cannabis can directly and indirectly affect the ECS.

In *Beyond Cannabis*, I will explore the synergistic use and potential health benefits of plant compounds, including polyphenols, terpenes, and dietary cannabinoids, other than the cannabis plant. I propose that combining terpenes, polyphenols, and dietary cannabinoids (not from *Cannabis sativa*) provides a "super additive" anti-inflammatory effect that we can apply use to combat autoimmune, metabolic, neurodegenerative, and other inflammatory diseases.

I will discuss some of the latest findings from research conducted on natural products derived from plants (and foods) other than cannabis that target proteins within the ECS. For instance, you will discover that Beta Caryophyllene (BCP) in copaiba balsam, and the alkyl amides in Echinacea are both direct CB2 (cannabinoid receptor 2) agonists and how the polyamides in chocolate block hydrolytic enzymes that control endocannabinoid levels, to name a few examples.

The fact that we can intentionally manipulate our ECS by choosing how we interact with it is as fascinating as it is promising. Indeed, understanding the profound anti-inflammatory effects offered by gently stimulating the ECS with diet, herbal medicine, and other lifestyle choices can bring tremendous relief to those struggling with chronic inflammation and immune dysfunction. And the more we understand the synergistic use of these compounds (in plants and through their essential oils, polyphenols, and dietary cannabinoids), the more we can personalize combinations to shore up our defenses and improve our health.

HEALING AT THE LEVEL OF GENE TRANSCRIPTION
As we live longer, regulating sugar, fat, and inflammatory gene expression has become a top priority for healthy aging and for controlling and even halting chronic disease.

Given that many experience an over-expression of inflammatory genes, as seen in metabolic syndrome and autoimmune and neurodegenerative diseases, we need to apply the most advanced anti-inflammatory strategies to effectively offset inflammation and immune reactions. This includes using polyphenols, terpenes, and dietary cannabinoids that specifically target key anti-inflammatory gene transcription factors NFKB (Nuclear Factor KB) and PPAR's (Peroxisome Proliferator-Activated Receptors) associated with improved insulin signaling, immune modulation, carbohydrate and fat metabolism.

Otherwise, we are left with using ulcer-inducing NSAIDs, steroids, cholinesterase inhibitors, biologics, thiazolidinedione, anti-depressants and anti-anxiety agents for the rest of our lives.

REGULATING INFLAMMATORY GENE EXPRESSION

Epigenetic studies show that we have the power to affect our genetic expression by changing the environmental signals that trigger the over-expressions of inflammatory genes. According to the latest science, environmental signals (including food, botanicals, and air quality) have the power to inform the promoter region genes that translate genotype into phenotype. Knowing how to manipulate these environmental inputs can therefore result in some powerful health benefits.

Nutrigenomics is an emerging science that studies the role of phytonutrients as a treatment for inflammation and immune modulation. By personalizing combinations of the most potent dietary cannabinoids, polyphenols and terpenes that act on CB2, NFKB and PPAR's we can experience the benefits of nutrigenomics.

Research on cannabidiol (CBD) has helped elucidate the mechanisms through which cannabis impacts our physiology. The surprise about cannabidiol (CBD) is that this non-psychoactive component of cannabis exerts its effects not on cannabinoid receptors, but on the precise metabolic and inflammatory regulation points or gene transcription factors that we will explore, namely PPARs and NFKB.

It is through these same exact pathways that many common foods and medicinal herbs exhibit similar anti-inflammatory effects to CBD, largely due to the chemical constituents that act on NFKB and PPARs (PPARα and PPARγ) namely, terpenes, phytocannabinoids and polyphenols.

The potent anti-inflammatory and therapeutic effects that come with specific combinations of these compounds have been demonstrated for centuries via the enduring success of traditional herbal medicine. All medicinal herbs have marked therapeutic effects on their own and synergistic effects when combined in remedies. In effect, plant foods and botanicals containing these potent compounds exert their impact through PPAR interaction, NFKB inhibition as well as improved histone and DNA methylation. This results in a less inflammation, and the greatest possible health.

NFKB and PPARs
NFKB (nuclear factor KB) and PPAR (Peroxisome Proliferator-Activated Receptors) pathways are important therapeutic targets for inflammation and metabolic dysfunction (i.e., glucose and lipid dysregulation).

Most health conscious people are familiar with polyphenols, flavonoids, antioxidants, vitamins, minerals, and omega-3 fatty acids to maintain health and prevent disease. What's becoming increasingly clear is how these compounds exert beneficial effects not only via PPAR activation but also through interactions with the NFKB system.

NFKB is a protein that acts like a switch to turn inflammation either "on" or "off" when cells sense "danger" in the form of infections, emotional, and/or metabolic stress. If this protein group is over-active, it will continually produce the inflammation response where none is needed. Knowing how to counteract inflammatory gene expression once the NFKB switch has been turned "on," can help decrease inflammation while you treat and heal any chronic disease.

Obviously, getting rid of infections and other stressors is the first step in preventing NFKB from turning inflammation "on" in the first place. Yet, since inflammation is the common denominator in all chronic diseases, it makes sense to use natural agents that inhibit the over-expression of NFKB. That over-expression may result in feeling inflamed, lethargic, and lacking in mental clarity, to name a few examples.

Polyphenols, terpenes and dietary cannabinoids that inhibit NFKB

We now know that safe and effective NFKB inhibitors are available from foods, herbal medicine and essential oils. The following NFKB inhibitors are promising candidates for both the prevention and treatment of chronic inflammation. Keep in mind going forward that many of these also act on the PPAR receptors and some, like Beta-Caryophyllene also acts directly on the CB2 receptor.

Common Natural NFKB Inhibitors	
• Allicin in garlic	• Sulphoraphane (found in cruciferous vegetables like broccoli)
• Curcumin in turmeric	• Vitamins A, C, E
• ECGC and theanine in green tea	• Berberine in barberry, scutellaria baicalensis, and goldenseal
• Gingkolides in gingko biloba	• N-acetylcysteine (NAC)
• Melatonin	• S-adenosyl-methionine (SAMe)
• Quercetin in onions, leeks	• Lipoic acid in organ meat, spinach
• Resveratrol in grapes, wine	• Zinc in oysters
• Silymarin in milk thistle	• EPA/DHA in fish oil
• Carnosol in rosemary	• Gingerols in ginger
• Beta-Caryophyllene in copaiba	• Myrcene in lavender and frankincense essential oil
• Limonene in lemon, orange and grapefruit essential oils	• Alpha-pinene in pine, sage and eucalyptus essential oils

PPARs

When it was discovered that THC and other cannabinoids were not the only plant compounds that can affect the ECS, the story about other modulatory partners began to include PPAR agonists (Davis, MP, 2014).

Peroxisome Proliferator-Activated Receptors (PPARs) are nuclear transcription factors (like NFKB) that regulate antioxidant and anti-inflammatory pathways. There are 3 main PPARs studied to date, each one possessing distinct tissue distribution and function in the regulation of energy metabolism.

In general, PPARα promotes fatty acid (FA) catabolism,

PPARγ enhances insulin sensitivity and lipid storage while PPARδ (also referred to as PPAR-β) changes the body's fuel preference from glucose to lipids and suppresses macrophage-derived inflammation. Recently it was discovered that all three PPARs PPARα, PPARγ *and* PPARδ are found on macrophages and when activated, decrease TNF alpha and IL6 (associated with inflammation) (Wang. 2014). These findings suggest the anti-inflammatory and immune modulating benefits of PPAR activation in many chronic diseases.

PPAR activation
It is now known that PPAR activation is linked to the suppression of pro-inflammatory genes via an interference with the NFKB signaling pathway. Once PPARs are activated by hormones, terpenes, fatty acids, and/or polyphenols they bind to nuclear DNA to promote or prevent transcription of specific genes involved in energy homeostasis, lipid uptake and metabolism, insulin sensitivity, and other metabolic functions. Since each of these mechanisms overlaps with observed effects in the ECS like alterations in energy, lipid and glucose metabolism, hunger and satiety, inflammation and pain, we must consider PPAR modulation as a means to regulating the ECS.

The ability of certain plants and compounds to modulate PPAR's has promising therapeutic implications, particularly with respect to autoimmunity, neurodegenerative and metabolic disorders. Our ability to access natural PPAR modulating ligands through foods and herbs (see below) offers us a much safer alternative in comparison to the currently available synthetic drugs for these diseases.

PPARγ

PPARγ expression is found in adipose tissue, colonic epithelia, macrophages, and endothelium, as well as the kidney, liver, and small intestine. Of all the PPARs, PPARγ improves insulin sensitivity to balance glucose in the blood. While Big Pharma has been selling drugs for type II Diabetes that act on this receptor for years, you may be interested to know that there are a number of herbs (such as Gymnema sylvestrae) and foods that possess natural PPARγ ligands. Personalized combinations of these compounds are known to increasing insulin sensitivity.

Some potent constituents in common foods that act on PPARγ include the catechism in green tea, tocotrienols in palm oil, 2'-Hydroxy chalcone in cinnamon, Psi-baptigenin and hesperidin in red clover, resveratrol in grapes and wine, astaxanthin in microalgae and crustaceans, carnosic acid in sage and rosemary, rosmarinic acid in marjoram, EPA/DHA in fish oil, flavonoids in licorice, conjugated linoleic acid in meat, carvocrol in thyme oil, quercetin in dill, bay leaves, and oregano, 6-shogaol in ginger roots and the triterpenes in ginseng.

PPARγ agonists have also been shown to be regulators of brain inflammation and oxidative stress (Bernardo. 2006, Collino. 2006). The majority of studies have shown that PPARγ agonists inhibit the expression of inflammatory mediators such as inducible nitric oxide synthase, by antagonizing activation of transcription factors such as NFKB. Since PPARγ is also suspected to be a neuroprotective agent (Yu. 2008), it would make sense to include natural ligands that activate PPARγ in cases of epilepsy, neuro-inflammation, and Alzheimer.

PPARα

PPAR-α expression is relatively high in hepatocytes, enterocytes, vascular and immune cell types such as monocytes/macrophages, endothelial cells, smooth muscle cells, lymphocytes, non-neuronal cells like microglia and astroglia and mainly regulates genes involved in the metabolism of lipids and lipoproteins (Fruchart. 2009).

Studies about PPARα also show that like PPARδ/PPAR-β, and PPARγ, this transcription factor is expressed in macrophages, and that PPARα agonists inhibit animal models of autoimmune conditions such as MS (Racke et al., 2006). Since microalgae (e.g. astaxanthin), olive oil, EPA and DHA are known PPARα ligands (binding molecules), it makes sense to consider these in a personalized program for autoimmune disease.

The fatty acid family N-acylethanolamides (including oleamides in chocolate and N-palmitoylethanolamide [PEA]) also bind directly to PPARα. PPARα is the transcription factor that regulates the breakdown of our internally produced lipid ligands called endocannabinoids. As we shall soon discover, the levels of our internally produced cannabinoids (aka endocannabinoids) anandamide and 2AG, can be manipulated by activating PPARα. Since anandamide is degraded by the fatty acid amide hydrolase (FAAH), enzyme inhibitors of FAAH will lead to elevated anandamide levels and can be pursued for therapeutic use. By suppressing the FAAH enzyme, polyamides may not only help increase anandamide levels, but also keep PPARα activated, which may result in enhanced PPARα transmission. PPARα activation in and of itself is considered anti-inflammatory (Costa, 2012).

PPARδ aka PPAR-β

PPARδ/PPAR-β is an important regulator of lipid metabolism and energy balance in adipose tissue, skeletal muscle, and the heart and is highly expressed in the colon, small intestine, liver and keratinocytes, as well as in heart, spleen, skeletal muscle, lung, brain and thymus (Wright, et al., 2000). PPARδ/PPAR-β, known to suppress macrophage derived inflammation, has also been shown to inhibit Th1 and Th17 responses (Kanakasabai, et al., 2010).

It is interesting to note that PPARδ/PPAR-β is mostly found in keratinocytes which constitutes about 90% of the cells found in the epidermis. Keratinocytes form tight junctions with the nerves of the skin and produce anti-inflammatory mediators such as IL-10 and TGF-β. This may prove to one of the mechanisms through which many herbal medicines may influence the ECS topically and also one of the ways in which bodywork may influence the ECS i.e. through mechanical stimulation via the keratinocytes.

Herbal Medicine and PPARS

Many natural remedies and herbal extracts have been studied for their effect on suppressing NFKB, the key regulator of inflammation, as well as on peroxisome proliferator-activated receptors PPARs.

Many herbs in Traditional Chinese Medicine (TCM) have been shown to not only inhibit TNF-α-induced NFKB activation, but also to act as agonists toward the peroxisome proliferator-activated receptors PPARs. In one study, 43% of Chinese Herbal Medicines showed NFKB inhibitory and 50% PPARα and PPARγ activating effects (Rozema et al., 2012). Traditional herbs excel in the treatment of chronic conditions by working not only on PPAR's and NFKB, but also on improved DNA methylation. The takeaway is that you may want to consider using specific botanicals from the Chinese Herbal Medicine pharmacy for your chronic inflammatory, autoimmune or neurodegenerative condition.

Reviewing the literature on this subject makes it clear that the herbal compounds that contain terpenes, polyphenols, and/or phytocannabinoids all exert their anti-inflammatory effects at the precise intervention point by interacting with gene transcription factors (PPARs and NFKB). In effect, these herbal compounds can regulate glucose and lipid metabolism while also keeping the inflammation switch turned "off." Since many of the proven effects of these constituents are associated with their ability to control PPAR receptors, it makes sense to incorporate these into an anti-inflammatory diet.

THE ENDOCANNABINOID SYSTEM (ECS) DEFINED

"Metaphorically the endocannabinoid system represents a microcosm of psychoneuroimmunology or mind-body medicine." John McPartland

The endocannabinoid system (ECS) was originally thought to be comprised of cannabinoid receptors (CB1 and CB2), two lipid-signaling molecules known as the endocannabinoids anandamide (AEA) and 2-arachidonoylglycerol (2-AG) and the enzymes MAGL and FAAH, (that break down AEA and 2AG). More current thinking, however, deems the ECS to include the orphan receptor GPR55 and arachidonic acid-derived ligands, which target other receptors such TRPV1 and PPARγ (De Petrocellis and Di Marzo, 2010) along with other ligands (e.g. polyphenols and terpenes) used to regulate endocannabinoid levels and activity at the receptors.

The main function of the endocannabinoid system is thought to be in neuromodulation i.e. controlling motor functions, cognition, emotional responses, homeostasis and motivation. However, in the periphery, the ECS is considered an important modulator of the autonomic nervous system, the immune system, and microcirculation (Nagarkatti. 2009). Given the broad reach of the ECS, knowing how to increase the tone of this system may prove to be your most powerful tool for halting many chronic diseases.

ENDOCANNABINOIDS AKA THE BODY'S CANNABINIOID SYSTEM

Endocannabinoids are the fatty acid substances produced in the body that activate cannabinoid receptors. N-arachidonylethanolamide (anandamide, AEA) and 2-arachidonoylglycerol (2-AG) are considered endocannabinoid ligands that are released from phospholipid precursors embedded in cell membranes.

Cannabinoids are the entire class of compounds that influence the cannabinoid receptors both in the central nervous system and the immune system. Ligands (binding molecules) for these receptors include both endocannabinoids that our body naturally produces and dietary cannabinoids aka phytocannabinoids (e.g. Beta-Caryophyllene, in copaiba, cloves, basil, rosemary, oregano, lavender, cinnamon, and black pepper).

While anandamide, 2-AG and their receptors CB1 and CB2, have been the most studied, the latest thinking about the entire ECS has expanded with the discovery of secondary receptors (PPAR's) that are now considered part of the endocannabinoid system. We are learning more about non-CB1 non-CB2 endocannabinoid receptors (PPARs), endocannabinoid-related molecules with little activity at CB1 and CB2 level, and new enzymes for the biosynthesis and degradation of these molecules (Di Marzo, 2009). As you shall soon discover, some of the precursors can be easily sourced through diet to increase endocannabinoid tone.

Anandamide

In 1992, Raphael Mechoulam of Hebrew University was the first to identify anandamide, the endogenous fatty acid ligand (arachidonoyl ethanolamine- AEA) that binds to the CB1 receptor. Anandamide, which is found in nearly all tissues of animals, is about as potent as THC at the CB1 receptor. (Grotenhermen, et al., 2005).

Anandamide mainly plays a role in the regulation of feeding behavior, memory and the neural generation of motivation and pleasure. Another important finding is that anandamide not only acts as a ligand for both cannabinoid receptors (CB1 and CB2) and vanilloid receptors (TRPV) that attenuate pain sensation (DiMarzo et al., 2002). Endogenous anandamide is generally present for a short amount of time due to the action of the enzyme FAAH which breaks it down into arachidonic acid and ethanolamine.

2-Arachidonoylglycerol (2-AG)

2-Arachidonoylglycerol (2 AG), the second endocannabinoid, was described by Shimon Ben-Shabat of Ben-Gurion University in 1994. 2AG is an endocannabinoid that stimulates the CB2 receptor, which is now well known for its anti-inflammatory effects. CB2 is the main receptor we will focus on due to its anti-inflammatory and immune modulating effects.

While you will soon discover other plants compounds that stimulate the cannabinoid receptors, one of the most important takeaways here is that our bodies naturally produce these feel-good, self-regulating compounds anandamide (after the Sanskrit word for "bliss") that binds to the CB1 receptor as well as anti-inflammatory compounds like 2AG that binds to the CB2 receptor.

Endocannabinoids, Inflammation and The Immune System

We now know that the endocannabinoid system, especially the CB2 receptor, is involved in immune regulation and neuroprotection. The mechanisms of immune regulation by endocannabinoids include modulation of immune response, decrease in cytokines, induction of apoptosis in immune cells, and the downregulation of innate and adaptive immune response (Hicks, 2015). Due to the distribution on CB2 receptors in the immune system, CB2 receptor stimulation with cannabinoids may prove important in autoimmune conditions.

CB2 receptor stimulation was shown to affect B-cell differentiation, and agonists (ligands that bind to CB2 receptors) were shown to suppress the proliferation of both B and T lymphocytes (Nargarkati et al., 2009). CB2 receptors stimulation can also suppress the activity of NK cells, which are the cells that lead to cell destruction and the proliferation of autoimmune diseases and neural inflammation. (Hicks, 2015).

Cannabinoid receptor stimulation has also been shown to affect the number and function of T cells, B cells, natural killer cells, dendritic cells, microglia and macrophages in rodents and humans (Croxford and Yamamura, 2005).

Cannabinoid receptor stimulation can also suppress the production of pro-inflammatory cytokines including TNFα,

Il-1β, IL-2, IL-6, IL-12 and IFN-γ, as well as cell proliferation, antigen presentation and trafficking into inflamed tissues (Rieder *et al.*, 2010). Because the CB2 receptor is primarily expressed on immune cells many of these effects are mediated via the CB2 receptor (Mackie, 2005).

This is noteworthy for people with untamed immune cells in the case of autoimmune arthritis or other autoimmune reactions. Learning how to shore up endocannabinoid levels and stimulate the CB2 receptor may be the key to shutting down inflammation and balancing the immune system.

Since the CB2 receptor does not cause psychoactivity and is associated with decreased inflammation, insulin signaling/sensitivity, satiety, and energy balance, this receptor is the key target for its potential to treat chronic disease. This research suggests that the use of CB2 receptor ligands, sourced from common foods and plants other than cannabis, may be a promising treatment for conditions ranging from Alzheimer to metabolic syndrome to autoimmune disease.

The endocannabinoid system also provides antioxidant, anti-inflammatory and neuronal protection. (Jackson et al., 2005). Recently other endocannabinoids and related *N*-acylethanolamines (NAEs) like PEA palmitoylethanolamide and OEA oleoylethanolamide have emerged as important regulators of metabolism and inflammation (Di Marzo et al., 2008). PEA palmitoylethanolamide is considered anti-inflammatorey while OEA oleoylethanolamide has appetite stimulating effects. PPARα activation is responsible for mediating the anti-inflammatory actions of palmitoylethanolamide (Lo Verme J., 2005).

Endocannabinoid Effect on Neurotransmitters
Although they have a similar role to neurotransmitters, endocannabinoids differ in that they use what has been referred to as retrograde signaling. That is, they are not stored in vesicles like neurotransmitters but are instead available in the cell membranes where they are synthesized as needed.

"Within the central nervous system, the endocannabinoid system acts as a negative feedback mechanism to dampen synaptic release of classic neurotransmitters" (McPartland, 2008). Endocannabinoids are thought to regulate neurotransmitter release e.g. dopamine, serotonin, acetylcholine and gaba. This is likely how they exert their impact on mood.

DIETARY CANNABINOIDS AKA PHYTOCANNABINOIDS

Dietary cannabinoids, aka phytocannabinoids have been defined as plant-derived natural products capable of either interacting directly with cannabinoid receptors or sharing chemical similarity with cannabinoids or both. (Gertsch, et al., 2010). In light of this definition, phytocannabinoids include *N*-acylethanolamines like PEA palmitoylethanolamide, OEA oleoylethanolamide, as well as terpene/dietary cannabinoid such as Beta-Caryophyllene (BCP) in common plants and their essential oils e.g. black pepper, cloves, cinnamon, hops and copaiba. All of these compounds work by either combining directly with a cannabinoid receptor (e.g. BCP that targets the CB2 receptor) or inhibiting the enzyme FAAH (e.g. polyamides in chocolate which activate PPARα), which in turn increases the levels of endocannabinoids, such as anandamide, produced by the body.

Since the ECS plays a major role in pain, immune function, inflammation, and hunger, we may experience illness when the ECS is out of balance. Because we now know that plant compounds can affect the ECS by interacting directly with cannabinoid receptors, inhibiting the enzymes that break down endocannabinoids, and/or influencing the availability of phospholipid precursors used to synthesize endocannabinoids (Gertsch et al., 2010), it makes sense to add in dietary cannabinoids to support and tone the ECS.

Dietary cannabinoids can stimulate the ECS and we can use dietary intervention as an effective way of supporting the ECS and getting it into a more balanced state that supports and promotes healing. Knowing how to shore up the ECS, including how to stimulate CB2 naturally with BCP, will go a long way to decreasing inflammation and regulating immune function.

Cannabinoid Receptors
The term "cannabinoid receptors" was coined after it was recognized that THC from cannabis interacted with specific human receptors. Because we have endocannabinoid receptors in every cell of the body, we respond to anything similar from an exogenous source (e.g, Beta-Caryophyllene in copaiba or even the stimulate from acupuncture needles) that stimulates the cannabinoid receptors (CB2) in the immune system.

While there is now evidence of even more receptors, we will focus on CB1 and CB2, the two main types of cannabinoid receptors, with CB2 being the main (non-psychoactive) target for decreasing inflammation and modulating the immune system.

As we move forward in our understanding of the endocannabinoid system, please consider how natural CB2 receptor stimulation along with foods that activate PPARs and turn off NFKB, can be a powerful combination for inflammation and autoimmune disease. Knowing how to combine these in a personalized program may lead to some remarkable results. For now, let's understand more about our endocannabinoid receptors and how gentle stimulation adds to overall endocannabinoid tone.

ENDOCANNABINOID RECEPTORS

Although there is a lot of overlap, CB1 receptors are mainly located in the brain and central nervous system while CB2 receptors are found more in the immune system. That being said, we need to pay close attention to supporting CB2 pathways for those with autoimmune reactions. Let's now consider the location and function of these receptors and the plants that might increase their tone.

CANNABINOID RECEPTOR TYPE 1 (CB1)

Because CB1 expression is found throughout the brain and central nervous system, in the basal ganglia, and the limbic system, including in the hippocampus and cerebellum, it has an influence on both excitatory and inhibitory neuronal circuits that regulate movement, memory, learning, cognition, neuroendocrine output, appetite, nausea, the regulation of body temperature, pain, and immune system modulation (Croxford and Yamamura, 2005). This broad ability to regulate synaptic neurotransmission means that stimulating CB1 has great potential in treating a wide range of conditions.

PLANTS THAY HAVE DIRECT ACTION ON THE CB1 RRECEPTOR (CB1)

The most well-known plant constituent shown to interact directly with the CB1 receptor includes *Delta*-9-tetrahydrocannabinol (Δ^9-THC, THC) from cannabis sativa. THC mimics the action of anandamide, binding to the CB1 cannabinoid receptors in the brain and central nervous system, where it produces its psychoactive effects. The Kava plant contains yangonin, a constituent that also acts as a ligand to stimulate the CB1 receptor (DiMarzo 2012).

These plants add to the list of promising natural compounds that stimulate the CB1 receptor.

CANNABINOID RECEPTOR TYPE 2 (CB2)

CB2 receptors are mainly found mainly the immune system (in lymphocytes, macrophages, NK and microglial cells), but also found in the cerebral cortex in the orbital, visual, motor, and auditory areas as well as in the hippocampus, the corpus callosum, cerebellum, brain stem, and pineal gland. Given their global status throughout the body, CB2 receptors can modify brain function and immune function. I imagine researchers will soon discover the link between music and visualization and ECS tone. Interestingly, CB2 receptors are also found in the enteric nervous system, which modulates gastrointestinal contractility. (Duncan et al., 2008). In cases of immune, brain and gut issues, using natural CB2 agonists like Beta-Caryophyllene, may provide powerful relief.

PLANTS THAY HAVE DIRECT ACTION ON THE CB2 RECEPTOR

There are an increasing number of natural products that target the CB2 receptor. Plant products reported to target the CB2 receptor include rutamarin in Ruta graveolens L. (Rollinger et al., 2009) and 3, 3'-diindolylmethane (DIM) commonly found in cruciferous vegetables. There are also many common plants that contain Beta-Caryophyllene which also stimulates the CB2 receptor. Read on to understand more about the dual identity of Beta-Caryophyllene as both a terpene and dietary cannabinoid.

THE MOST PROMISING CB2 RECEPTOR STIMULANTS

Remember that CB2 is the main target for regulating inflammation, modulating the immune system, and improving endocannabinoid tone. Beta-Caryophyllene (BCP) is a sesquiterpene that also has the ability to bind to the CB2 receptor. BCP binds to anti-inflammatory CB2 cannabinoid receptors and therefore also categorized as a cannabinoid. BCP found in cannabis as well as many other herbs and common foods, is considered both a terpene and a dietary cannabinoid due to its ability to act directly on CB2.

Low Dose Beta-Caryophyllene Therapy
The fact that BCP is found in large amounts in the essential oils of commonly used herbs and spices (including cloves, basil, rosemary, oregano, lavender, cinnamon, copaiba and black pepper) suggests that low dose Beta-Caryophyllene stimulation of the CB2 receptor is available via diet and aromatherapy. In fact, it's the BCP content in many herbs and essential oils that are responsible for the anti-inflammatory and neuro-hormonal modulating effects of these herbs and oils. (Bahi et al., 2014).

Since BCP does not bind to the CB1 receptor and therefore does not exert psychoactive effects, it has massive potential for treating pain, inflammation, autoimmune disease, and more. One human study showed that BCP selectively binds to the CB2 receptor and inhibits LPS-stimulated TNFα and IL-1b expression in peripheral blood

(Gertsch et al., 2008). Another study found that β-Caryophyllene activation of both CB2 and PPARγ pathways; has the beneficial effect of reducing neuro-inflammatory response in the treatment of Alzheimer disease (Cheng, 2014). Anxiolytic, and antidepressant, and anti-alcoholism effects have also been reported (Bahi et al., 2014).

BCP has been shown to exert significant anti-inflammatory effects in mice. BCP from copaiba balsam was shown to be neuroprotective (Santos, 2012). BCP is even an FDA-approved food additive and has been termed the "first dietary cannabinoid." (Gertsch, 2010). Because BCP targets CB2 receptors without any psych activity, BCP offers an effective anti-inflammatory/analgesic without any alteration in perception or motor skills. Given the multiple benefits of BCP, we should consider it for inflammatory, autoimmune, and/or metabolic disorders.

Some alkyl amides from the *Echinacea* plant have also been shown to interact with the human CB2 receptor. Notably, the CB2 receptor-binding *N*-alkyl amides from Echinacea shows similar anti-inflammatory effects as anandamide (e.g. inhibition of TNF-α). Like anandamide and CBD, *N*-alkyl amides also target PPARγ, a nuclear transcription protein that turns off TNF alpha and IL6, which explains their effect on inflammation. (Gertsch et al., 2010).

POLYPHENOLS AND THE ENDOCANNABINOID SYSTEM

Polyphenols are known to interact with multiple protein binding sites. Since most cannabinoid receptor ligands are highly lipophilic, hydrophilic polyphenols are considered atypical or indirect CB ligands. To date, studies on polyphenols and the ECS have indicated that ECGC in green tea, curcumin in turmeric, and trans-resveratrol in red wine were found to be weak CB receptor agonists and instead shown to exert their impact through PPAR activation and altering enzymes like MAGL and FAAH which contributes to overall ECS tone. Other indirect ligands are listed in this chart.

INDIRECT CANNABINOID RECEPTOR LIGANDS

Name	Origin	CB receptor affinity	Function	In vivo efficacy	Other targets (ECS)	References
N-acylethanolamines	Widespread in plants	No affinity	FAAH inhibitors Indirect cannabimimetics	Validated in CB_1 and CB_2 KO mice	GPR55	Maurelli et al., 1995; Di Tomaso et al., 1996; Di Marzo, 2008
Salvinorin A	Salvia divinorum	Insignificant affinity to CB receptors	Indirect cannabimimetic effects at CB1 (mechanism unknown)	No data	KOP agonist	Capasso et al., 2008; Fichna et al., 2009;
Pristimerin	Relatively widespread in the Celastraceae	No data	Potent reversible MAGL inhibitor (IC50 value <100 nM)	No data	No data	King et al., 2009
Kaempferol	Widespread in plants	No affinity	FAAH inhibitor (IC_{50} value <1 µM)	No data	No data	Thors et al., 2007; 2008
Trans-resveratrol	Relatively widespread in plants (e.g. Vitis vinifera L.)	Insignificant affinity	Insignificant effects	No data	No data	Prather et al., 2009
Curcumin	Curcuma spp.	Insignificant affinity	Insignificant effects	No data	No data	Prather et al., 2009
Epigallocatechin-3-O-gallate	Relatively widespread in plants (e.g. Camellia sinensis L.)	Insignificant affinity	No data	No data	No data	Korte et al., 2010

ECS, endocannabinoid system; FAAH, fatty acid amide hydrolase; MAGL, monoacylglycerol lipase.

DIRECT CANNABINOID RECEPTOR LIGANDS

Name	Origin	CB receptor affinity	Function	In vivo efficacy	Other targets (ECS)	References
Δ^9-THC	Cannabis sativa L.	Non-selective CB_1 and CB_2 affinity (K_i values <50 nM) (human)	Partial agonist G_i/o Inhibition by SR141716 and SR144528	Validated in CB_1 and CB_2 KO mice	GPR55 PPARs Different ion channels	Mechoulam, 1986; Pertwee, 2006
N-alkylamide	Echinacea spp.	Selective CB_2 affinity (K_i value <100 nM) (human)	Parial agonist $[Ca^{2+}]_i$ Inhibition by SR144528	No data	PPAR-γ Inhibition of AEA transport Partial FAAH inhibition	Raduner et al., 2006; Chicca et al., 2009
β-caryophyllene	Widespread in plants	Selective CB_2 affinity (K_i value <200 nM) (human)	Full agonist G_i/o $[Ca^{2+}]_i$	Validated in CB_2KO mice	No data	Gertsch et al., 2008
Falcarinol	Relatively widespread in Apiaceae (e.g. Daucus carota L.)	Non-selective CB_1 affinity (K_i value <1 µM) (human)	CB_1 receptor-selective inverse (covalent) agonist Inhibition of AEA/WIN55212-2	No data	No data	Leonti et al., 2010
Rutamarin	Ruta graveolens L.	Selective CB_2 affinity (K_i value <10 µM) (human)	No data	No data	No data	Rollinger et al., 2009
DIM 3,3-diindolylmethane metabolite from indole-3-carbinol	Relatively widespread in the Brassica genus	Selective CB_2 affinity (K_i value ≅1 µM) (human)	Partial agonist at CB_2 receptor	No data	No data	Yin et al., 2009

Δ^9-THC is shown as the major phytocannabinoid from Cannabis sativa L. but there are several other structurally related cannabinoids that interact with CB receptors.

Δ^9-THC, Δ^9-tetrahydrocannabinol; DIM, 3,3'-diindolylmethane; ECS, endocannabinoid system; FAAH, fatty acid amide hydrolase; PPAR, peroxisome proliferator-activated protein. Referenced from Gertsch, J., Pertwee, R. G. and Di Marzo, V. (2010), Phytocannabinoids beyond the *Cannabis* plant – do they exist?. British Journal of Pharmacology, 160: 523–529. doi: 10.1111/j.1476-5381.2010.00745.x

POLYPHENOLS

Every person with inflammation, from diabetes to mild arthritis to a full-blown autoimmune disease, is searching for the perfect balance of food and plant compounds that decrease inflammation and bring relief. The good news is that there are about 8000 compounds with antioxidant properties in the polyphenol family, all with impressive health benefits. Since it is becoming clear that polyphenols also influence the ECS via PPAR activation and NFKB suppression, it makes sense to consider them in a program to support your ECS.

There are many other dietary choices that show similarities in influencing the ECS. Trans-resveratrol, curcumin and ECGC (in green tea), like cannabidiol act indirectly on the ECS via PPAR activation vs. cannabinoid receptor activation. Given this information, it seems appropriate to include other PPAR (and NFKB) ligands from polyphenols that have the potential to change gene transcription. Most of these ligands include common flavonoids (part of the polyphenol family) that can be found in our diet. While it's obvious that polyphenols are found in abundance in nature, our next step is to hunt, gather, and be efficient with the active ingredients to yield significant results.

POLYPHENOLS

Polyphenol Type	Dietary Source			Pharmacological Activity References
Phenolic Acids	Coffee (caffeic acid) Tea (gallic acid)			Anti-oxidative properties, cardio-protective properties associated with an enhanced anti-atherogenic function of HDL. (Uto-Kondo et al. 2010)
Lignans	Flax Strawberries Apricots Sesame seeds Broccoli Kale Cabbage Soy			Reduce inflammation, improve blood sugar, protect against heart disease and breast cancer. (Adlercreutz H. et al 2007 and Saarinen NM, et al. 2007)
Flavonoids Categories: Flavonols Flavan-3-ols Flavones Flavonones Isoflavones Anthocyanidins	**Fruits:** Apples Apricots Blackberries Blueberries Cherries Chokeberries Citrus Cranberries Currants Dates Elderberries Gooseberries Grapes Kiwi Lemon Ligonberries Limes Mangoes Marionberries Nectarines Peaches Pears Plums Prunes Pomegranates Quinces Raspberries Rhubarb Raisins Strawberries	**Vegetables:** Artichokes Broccoli Cabbage Carrot Celery Eggplant Fennel Garlic Greens Kohlrabi Kale Leeks Onions Black Olives Green Olives Peppers Parsnips Peas Rutabagas Scallions Shallots Spinach Sweet potatoes Tomatoes Watercress	**Fruits:** Apples Apricots Blackberries Blueberries Cherries Chokeberries Citrus Cranberries Currants Dates Elderberries Gooseberries Grapes Kiwi Lemon Ligonberries Limes Mangoes Marionberries Nectarines Peaches Pears Plums Prunes Pomegranates Quinces Raspberries Rhubarb Raisins Strawberries	
Flavonols: Quercetin Kaempferol Myricetin	Onions Kale Leeks Broccoli Blueberries Bok Choy Napa Cabbage Green Tea Endive			Quercitin suppresses brain inflammation. (Dajas F. et al 2015) Myricetin protects cells from carcinogenic mutations, inhibits viral activity, and protect neurons from oxidative stress. (Devi KP, et al 2015) Kaempferol in all Brassica vegetables inhibits cancer,

		reduces heart disease risk, and has proven antimicrobial, neuroprotective, antidiabetic, anti-osteoporotic, anti-anxiety, pain-relieving, and anti-allergic properties. Calderón-Montaño JM, et al. *Chem*. 2011
Flavan-3-ols aka Flavanols: Catechins and Proanthocyanidins (aka condensed tannins)	Apricots Red wine Green tea Grapes Peaches Berries Pears Dark chocolate	Flavanols support vascular health, and exhibit anti-microbial, anti-carcinogen, and neuro-protective properties. (Cassidy A, et al 2015, Ponzo V, et al 2015, Wang D, et al 2012)
Flavones: Luteolin and Apigenin	Parsley Celery Green peppers Citrus Skin Chamomile Chysanthemum	Luteolin suppresses production of the inflammatory cytokines TNFα, IL-1b, and IL-6, actions that relate to a selective reduction in numbers of monocytes (Lee YS, et al 2015) Luteolin protects against retinal oxidative stress (Hytti M, et al 2015) Luteolin has neuroprotective effects Theoharides TC, et al 2015
Isoflavones and Phytoestrogens Genistein and Daidzein	Flax Red Clover	Phytoestrogens (plant-derived, estrogen-like molecules) modulate the immune system's inflammatory responses, reduce the risk of certain hormone-dependent cancers, and decrease the severity of osteoporosis. Isoflavone-induced inhibition of NFKB is the mechanism by which isoflavones reduce the invasiveness of breast cancer and increase programmed cell death in various human cancer cell lines. (Uifalean A, et al 2015)
Flavanones	Citrus Mint Tomato	Cardio-protective, anti-inflammatory, anti-hypertensive, may improve insulin sensitivity. (Cassidy A, et al 2015, Ponzo V, et al 2015, Wang D, et al 2012)
Anthocyanidins	Berries Cherries Grapes Red cabbage Eggplant	Neuroprotective, anti-inflammatory, pain relieving. Flavanols support vascular health, and exhibit anti-microbial, anti-carcinogen, and neuro-protective properties. (Cassidy A, et al 2015, Ponzo V, et al 2015, Wang D, et al 2012)

ENDOCANNABINOID DEFICIENCY SYNDROME

Since cannabinoid receptors and their endogenous lipid ligands were discovered via research on *Cannabis sativa*, scientists started to define the regulatory function of our internally produced endo-CA cannabinoids (or lack thereof).

Endocannabinoids are responsible for regulating many physiological functions by acting as anti-inflammatory and neuro-hormonal modulators. Human studies suggest that endocannabinoid deficiency syndrome may be the hidden etiology in migraine, fibromyalgia, irritable bowel syndrome, schizophrenia, migraine, multiple sclerosis, Huntington's, Parkinson's, anorexia, and chronic motion sickness. (Russo et al, 2010).

Research has demonstrated alterations in the endocannabinoid system in chronic pain (Kaufmann et al., 2009) and in psychiatric patients (Koethe et al., 2007). Some studies show that serum levels of endocannabinoids are reduced in both depressed patients (Hill et al., 2009) and chronic pain patients (Fichna et al., 2013).

Interestingly, various polymorphisms of CB1 and CB2 receptors have been identified in patients with major depression and bipolar disorder (Mitjans et al., 2013). Similarly, genetic alterations in the CB1 receptor and the FAAH enzyme have also been identified in patients with pain associated with migraine, Parkinson's disease, and irritable bowel syndrome (Greenbaum et al., 2012).

Correcting endocannabinoid deficiency may be possible by enhancing endocannabinoid ligand synthesis, decreasing endocannabinoid ligand degradation, and augmenting or decreasing receptor density and function (Russo. 2009).

These findings support the idea of using small doses of dietary cannabinoids, polyphenols and terpenes regularly to support your ECS in cases of pain, inflammation, and mood disorders. Increasing endocannabinoid tone with dietary cannabinoids, terpenes, and polyphenols is equally promising for those with metabolic, inflammatory, and autoimmune disease. Studies show that when a person is deficient in endocannabinoids, certain fatty acids, terpenes, and polyphenols can be used to bolster endocannabinoid tone (Russo, 2011).

ENDOCANNABINOID TONE

Now that we know more about the protective effects of our ECS, our goal should be to increase cannabinoid tone. A great place to start is adding the potent members of the phyto-cannabinoid family (e.g., fatty acids, polyphenols and terpenes) to our diet. Many of the foods, herbs and essential oils presented in this guide work to increase endocannabinoid tone by acting either on PPAR's, NFKB, CB2 or all three (as in the case of Beta-Caryophyllene).

As we have seen, polyphenols act on PPAR's and NFKB to increase endocannabinoid tone. Dietary cannabinoids such as Beta-Caryophyllene increases endocannabinoid tone by stimulating the CB2 receptor and acting on PPARγ *and* NFKB. Studies also show that dietary levels of essential fatty acids affect the levels of anandamide and other endocannabinoids in the brain (Berger et al., 2001) thereby increasing endocannabinoid tone. EPA/DHA from fish oils also act on NFKB and PPAR's.

Other natural non-food therapies that have been proven effective for increasing endocannabinoid tone include meditation, yoga, acupuncture, massage and spinal manipulation (McPartland et al., 2008). For those with an endocannabinoid deficiency, regulating the levels of endocannabinoids with natural interventions, including dietary cannabinoids, terpenes, fatty acids, and polyphenols, as well as with acupuncture and other ways of communicating with the ECS, can be highly beneficial. All of these may go a long way to improving and maintaining endocannabinoid tone.

ACHIEVING THE ENTOURAGE EFFECT

Combining bioactive compounds such as terpenes, polyphenols, fatty acids, and cannabinoids can produce physiologic effects that have been referred to as "the entourage effect." When combined, terpenes in essential oils, polyphenols, and dietary cannabinoids produce a synergistic entourage effect on the ECS, which basically means that the therapeutic impact is more effective as a result. For example, pine essential oil contains a high amount of the terpene pinene, which is known not only for its potent anti-inflammatory effects but also for being an acetylcholinesterase inhibitor (due to 1, 8 cineole) used for improved memory and recall (McPartland and Pruitti, 1999). This would be a great addition to an anti-inflammatory diet that prioritizes PPARγ ligands (e.g. fish oil) for anyone suffering with neuro-inflammation, dementia or Alzheimer disease. By adding in specific anti-inflammatory foods and botanicals, you'll enhance the benefits of the treatment via the entourage effect.

As we have seen, polyphenols are the potent plant compounds that have the power to bind to and turn "off" nuclear transcription factors (which turn "off" inflammatory genes and regulate glucose and lipid metabolism). In this way they may act indirectly to regulate endocannabinoid tone. Dietary cannabinoids, like BCP, work by binding directly to the anti-inflammatory CB2 receptor and by activating PPARγ. Terpenes, which are abundant in essential oils, vegetables, and fruit, represent yet another group of compounds that can also affect the ECS.

TERPENES: THE ESSENTIAL OILS OF PLANTS

Terpenes are the volatile oils of plants that are considered the chief compounds in essential oils. The terpenes studied in cannabis are also found in many other plants and edible foods and have been used medicinally for centuries in the practice of aromatherapy.

Terpenes are pharmacologically versatile: they are lipophilic, interact with cell membranes, neuronal and muscle ion channels, neurotransmitter receptors, G-protein coupled receptors, second messenger systems and enzymes (Buchbauer, 2010). Terpenes have been shown to act as ligands to CB, NFKB and PPAR receptors, thereby halting inflammatory gene expression and being stellar candidates for any chronic disease. A review of the literature on aromatherapy suggests that endocannabinoid tone can also be enhanced by exogenous terpenes in essential oils.

The cannabis terpenoids: limonene, myrcene, α-pinene, linalool, β-caryophyllene, caryophyllene oxide, nerolidol and phytol are all phytotherapeutic agents in their own right and found in many other essential oils. "Terpenoids share a precursor with phytol-cannabinoids, and are all flavor and fragrance components common to human diets that have been designated Generally Recognized as Safe by the US Food and Drug Administration and other regulatory agencies. They display unique therapeutic effects that may contribute meaningfully to the entourage effects of cannabis-based medicinal extracts" (Russo, 2010).

Terpenes in the essential oils of plants have been shown to

interact with cannabinoid receptors in the immune, nervous, and gastrointestinal systems. Research also suggests that terpenes in combination with cannabinoids can alter the permeability of both cell membranes and the blood/brain barrier, causing phyto-cannabinoids to be more thoroughly absorbed (Russo. 2010).

It has been further pointed out that a combination of terpenoids and cannabinoids not only increase blood flow, enhance cortical activity, and have anti-inflammatory effects, but that cannabinoid-terpenoid interactions "could also produce synergy with respect to treatment of pain, inflammation, depression, anxiety, addiction, epilepsy, cancer, fungal, and bacterial infections." (Russo et al., 2011).

It is well known in the field of aromatherapy that diffused terpenes in essential oils (e.g, linalool in lavender and limonene in citrus) are proven allies for treating anxiety and depression, respectively. Studies show serotonenergic effects at the 5HT and 5 HT receptors by specific terpenes like linalool, which explains lavender oil mediated analgesia and mood alteration (Guzman, et al., 2015). Limonene, the terpene in lemon, sweet orange, and grapefruit has proven antidepressant and anti-anxiety effects. (Carvalho-Freitas and Costa, 2002; Pultirini A, et al., 2006. Komiya et al., 2006).

Some terpenes, like BCP in copaiba, act both directly on the cannabinoid receptors (CB2) and via PPARγ activation while other terpenes act indirectly via PPARα activation (e.g. pinene), which affects enzymes that inhibit the breakdown of e.g. acetylcholinesterase. Myrcene (the terpene in hops, frankincense and black pepper) and other terpenes are known to act as mixed agonist/antagonists of cannabinoid receptors, modulating the effects of anandamide and other endogenous ligands (McPartland et al., 2001).

Just as the selective use of high-torpedoed and high-phytocannabinoid-specific chemo types has become the target of medical marijuana research for disorders such as depression, anxiety, and dementia, we can also use precise essential oils, such as lavender plus citrus oils to lift anxiety and depression and pine oil for mental clarity, along with our dietary cannabinoids, polyphenols and fatty acids that help keep anandamide and 2AG in circulation. The terpene content in the essential oils (EO's) used in aromatherapy is what makes them so potent at a low dosage of a drop to a few drops/day.

The use of terpenes in aromatherapy adds to the entourage effect to lift depression, calm irritable nerves, and generally encourage a better state of mind. Some terpenes and phyto-cannabinoids like BCP can be applied topically for anti-inflammatory effects which may add to the entourage effect and increased endocannabinoid tone.

For more information on reproducing the entourage effect with essential oils, check out www.beyondcannabis.club.

Therapeutic terpenes can help you achieve the "Entourage Effect" with essential oils and aromatherapy.

Terpene	Essential Oils	Pharmacological Activity	Uses
Limonene (Monterpene)	Lemon Black Pepper Frankincense Orange Grapefruit Lemongrass	Potent AD/immunostimulant via inhalation (Komori et al., 1995) Anxiolytic (Carvalho-Freitas and Costa, 2002; Pultirini Ade et al., 2006 via 5-HT1A (Komiya et al., 2006) Apoptosis of breast cancer cells (Vigushin et al., 1998) Active against acne bacteria (Kim et al., 2008) Dermatophytes (Sanguinetti et al., 2007; Singh et al., 2010) Gastro-oesophageal reflux (Harries, 2010)	Treats Acid Reflux Anti-anxiety Antidepressant Antiseptic Immune-modulating
α-Pinene (Monoterpene)	Pine Orange Rosemary Sage Eucalyptus Galangal Cannabis Thyme Frankincense	Anti-inflammatory via PGE-1 (Gil et al, 1989) Bronchodilatory in humans (Falk et al., 1990) Acethylcholinesterase inhibitor, aiding memory (Perry et al., 2000)	Bronchodilator Aids Memory Anti-bacterial Anti-inflammatory
β-Myrcene (Monoterpene)	Hops Mango Bay Leaves Eucalyptus Lemongrass Parsley Verbena Thyme Black Pepper Myrrh Frankincense	Blocks inflammation via PGE-2 (Lorenzetti et al., 1991) Analgestic, antagonized by naloxone (Rao et al., 1990) Sedating, muscle relaxant, hypnotic (do Vale et al., 2002) Blocks hepatic carcinogenesis by aflatoxin (de Oliveira et al., 1997)	Sleep Aid Muscle Relaxant Anti-inflammatory
Linalool (Monoterpene)	Lavender Thyme Black Pepper Bergamot	Anti-anxiety (Russo, 2001) Sedative on inhalation in mice (Buchbauer et al., 1993) Local anesthetic (Re et al., 2000) Analgestic via adenosine A2A (Peana et al., 2006) Anticonvulsant/anti-glutamate (Elisabetsky et al., 1995) Potent anti-leishmanial (do Socorro et al., 2003)	Anesthetic Anticonvulsant Analgesic Anti-anxiety
β-Caryophyllene (Sesquiterpene)	Black Pepper Cloves Rosemary Cinnamon Oregano Thyme Basil Cannabis	AI via PGE-1 comparable phenylbutazone (Basile et al., 1988) Gastric cytoprotective (Tambe et al., 1996) Anti-malarial (Campbell et al., 1997) Selective CB2 agonist (100 nM) (Gertsch et al., 2008) Treatment of pruritus (Karsak et al., 2007) Treatment of addiction (Xi et al., 2010)	Anti-inflammatory Analgesic Protects the lining of the digestive tract Neuroprotective

Caryophyllene Oxide (Sesquiterpene)	Eucalyptus Lemon balm	Decreases platelet aggregation (Lin et al., 2003) Antifungal in onychomycosis comparable to Ciclopiroxolamine and sulconazole (Yang et al., 1999) Insecticidal/anti-feedant (Bettarini et al., 1993)	Antifungal Antiviral Antibacterial Antidepressant Anti-anxiety
Nerolidol (Sesquiterpene)	Orange Jasmine Lavender Tea Tree Lemongrass	Sedative (Binet et al., 1972) Skin penetrant (Cornwell and Barry, 1994) Potent antimalarial (Lopes et al., 1999, Rodrigues Goulart et al., 2004) Anti-leishmanial activity (Arruda et al., 2005)	Antianxiety Antifungal Antibacterial
Phytol (Diterpine)	Green tea Eucalyptus	Breakdown product of chlorophyll Prevents Vitamin A teratogenesis (Arnhold et al., 2002) ↑GABA via SSADH inhibition (Bang et al., 2002)	Antioxidant Antifungal Sleep aid Immune-modulating

5-HT, 5-hydroxytryptamine (serotonin); AD, antidepressant; AI, anti-inflammatory; CB1/CB2, cannabinoid receptor 1 or 2; GABA, gamma aminobutyric acid; PGE-1/PGE-2, prostaglandin E-1/prostaglandin E-2; SSADH, succinic semialdehyde dehydrogenase.
Gertsch, J., Pertwee, R. G. and Di Marzo, V. (2010), Phytocannabinoids beyond the *Cannabis* plant – do they exist?. British Journal of Pharmacology, 160: 523–529. doi: 10.1111/j.1476-5381.2010.00745.x

Promising phytocannabinoid and essential oil blends to achieve the entourage effect.

Essential Oil Blends	Essential Oil Terpene Profile	Uses
Body Buzz Frankincense Copaiba For topical use	Frankincese: a-pinene, a-phellandrene, limonene, B-myrcene, B-pinene, B-caryophyllene (BCP), p-cymene, Terpinen-4-ol, Verbenone, Sabinene, Linalool	Anti-inflammatory Anti-anxiety Pain reliever
	Copaiba: B-caryophyllene, pinene, sesquiterpenes, diterpenes, and terpenic acids	Anti-inflammatory BAntifungal Antiseptic
Calm Lavender Bergamot Best used with a diffuser	Lavender: a-pinene, limonene, camphor, linalool, caryophyllene, terpinen-4-ol	Sleep Aid Muscle Relaxant Anti-inflammatory
	Bergamot: a-pinene, myrcene, limonene, a-bergaptene, b-bisabolene, linalool, nerol, geraniol, and a-terpineol	Analgesic Antispasmodic Antibiotic Digestive
Mental Clarity Pine Eucalyptus Sage Best used with a diffuser	Pine: borneol, a and b-phallandrene, a and b-pinene and 3-carene	Antifungal Antiviral Antibacterial Antidepressant Anti-anxiety Aids Memory
	Eucalyptus: a-pinene, b-pinene, a-phellandrene, limonene, terpinen-4-ol	Bronchodilator Aids Memory Anti-bacterial Anti-inflammatory
	Sage: a-pinene, camphene, b-pinene, myrcene, limonene, 1,8-cineole, a-thujone, b-thujone, camphor, linalool, bornyl acetate and borneol.	Anti-inflammatory Antibacterial Antispasmodic
Uplifted Sweet Orange Lemon Grapefruit Best used with a diffuser	Sweet Orange: a-pinene, sabinene, myrcene, limonene, linalool, citronellal, neral and geranial	Anti-anxiety Antifungal Antibacterial
	Grapefruit: a-pinene, sabinene, myrcene, limonene, linalool, citronellal, neral, terpinen-4-ol, and geraniol	Anti-anxiety Antifungal Antibacterial Antidepressant
	Lemon: a-pinene, camphene, b-pinene, sabinene, myrcene, a-terpinene, linalool, b-bisabolene, limonene, trans-a-bergamotene, nerol and neral.	Treats Acid Reflux Anti-anxiety Antidepressant Antiseptic Immune-modulating

FINAL THOUGHTS

To halt chronic disease expression, we need to get a handle on the endocannabinoid system (ECS) and learn how best to interact with it. The research referenced in this guide demonstrates that our ECS is involved in multiple functions, and that modulating the activity of the ECS holds therapeutic promise in treating everything from diabetes, neuro-inflammation and autoimmunity, to mood and movement disorders. Given the growing number of pre-clinical studies and clinical trials revealing compounds that modulate the ECS, we should further explore novel therapeutic approaches for treating chronic inflammatory and/or autoimmune disease.

As you learn more about your own ECS, you will learn how best to support it with the food you eat, the air you breathe, and the treatments, including acupuncture, yoga, running, osteopathy, and other body work, for ultimate endocannabinoid tone. All of these treatments are encouraged for synergistic results. Add to the targeted polyphenols, essential oils and dietary cannabinoids that also regulate inflammatory, sugar, and lipid genes and you have a dynamic way of approaching all inflammatory and autoimmune disease processes.

For those looking to support the ECS, you may find that with the right inputs you may not need a medical marijuana prescription.

These are exciting times in this field of study. We are learning so much about the ECS. That being said, we are also just beginning to discover more information about something we've had all along, which is a sensitive protective layer in our body that needs nurturance to stay intact and support better health.

This guide was written for informational purposes only with the following references.

REFERENCES

Artmann A, Petersen G, Hellgren LI, Boberg J, Skonberg C, Nellemann C, Hansen SH, Hansen HS. "Influence of dietary fatty acids on endocannabinoid and N-acylethanolamine levels in rat brain, liver and small intestine." 2008.

Alejandro Cuevas et al. "Modulation of Immune Function by Polyphenols: Possible Contribution of Epigenetic Factors." Nutrients. 2013 Jul; 5(7): 2314–2332.

Bahi A., et al. "β-Caryophyllene, a CB2 Receptor agonist produces multiple behavioral changes relevant to anxiety and depression in mice." 2014

Banerjee SP, Snyder SH, Mechoulam R. "Cannabinoids: influence on neurotransmitter uptake in rat brain synaptosomes." J Pharmacol Exp Ther. 1975

Berger, Alvin; Crozier, Gayle; et al. "Anandamide and diet: Inclusion of dietary arachidonate and docosahexaenoate leads to increased brain levels of the corresponding N-acylethanolamines in piglets." *Proceedings of the National Academy of Sciences* **98** (11): 6402–6406. 15 May 2001.

Barrett, DA, Ho WS1, Randall MD. "Entourage' effects of N-palmitoylethanolamide and N-oleoylethanolamide on vasorelaxation to anandamide occur through TRPV1 receptors." Br J Pharmacol. 2008 Nov;155(6):837-46. doi: 10.1038/bjp.2008.324. Epub 2008 Aug 11.

Barnea, G, O'Donnell S, Mancia F, Sun X, Nemes A, Mendelsohn M, et al. "Odorant receptors on axon termini in the brain." Science. 2004

Baser, KHC, Buchbauer G, editors. "Aromatherapy with essential oils. In: Handbook of Essential Oils: Science, Technology, and Applications." Boca Raton, FL: CRC Press; 2010.

Basile, AC, Sertie JA, Freitas PC, Zanini AC. "Anti-inflammatory activity of oleoresin from Brazilian Copaifera." J Ethnopharmacol. 1988

Bernardo, Antonietta, and Luisa Minghetti. "PPAR-agonists as regulators of microglial activation and brain inflammation." Current Pharmaceutical Design 12.1 2006: 93-109.

Batista, PA, Werner MF, Oliveira EC, Burgos L, Pereira P, Brum LF, et al. "Evidence for the involvement of ionotropic glutamatergic receptors on the antinociceptive effect of (-)-linalool in mice." Neurosci Lett. 2008

Behav Brain Res. "Lemon oil vapor causes an anti-stress effect via modulating the 5-HT and DA activities in mice." 2006

Ben-Shabat S., Fride E, Sheskin T, Tamiri T, Rhee MH, Vogel Z, et al. "An entourage effect: inactive endogenous fatty acid glycerol esters enhance 2-arachidonoyl-glycerol cannabinoid activity." Eur J Pharmacol. 1998

Ben-Shabat S., Fride E, Sheskin T, Tamiri T, Rhee MH, Vogel Z, et al. "An entourage effect: inactive endogenous fatty acid glycerol esters enhance 2-arachidonoyl-glycerol cannabinoid activity." Eur J Pharmacol. 1998

Bisogno, T., Hanus L, De Petrocellis L, Tchilibon S, Ponde DE, Brandi I, et al. "Molecular targets for cannabidiol and its synthetic analogues: effect on vanilloid VR1 receptors and on the cellular uptake and enzymatic hydrolysis of anandamide." Br J Pharmacol. 2001; 134:845–852.

Boca Raton. "Aromatherapy with essential oils. In: Baser KHC, Buchbauer G, editors. Handbook of Essential Oils: Science, Technology, and Applications." FL: CRC Press; 2010.

Buchbauer G., Jirovetz L, Jager W, Plank C, Dietrich H. "Fragrance compounds and essential oils with sedative effects upon inhalation." J Pharm Sci. 1993

Carvahilo-Freitas MI, et al. "Anxiolytic and sedative effects of extracts and essential oil from Citrus aurantium. L." Biol Pharm Bull. 2002; 25:1629–1633. 2002.

Cheng Y1, Dong Z. "β-Caryophyllene ameliorates the Alzheimer-like phenotype in APP/PS1 Mice through CB2 receptor activation and the PPARγ pathway." Liu S. Pharmacology. 2014;94(1-2):1-12. Epub 2014 Aug 26.

Chinetti. G., et al. "Activation of proliferator-activated receptors alpha and gamma induces apoptosis of human monocyte-derived macrophages." Biol Chem. 1998 Oct 2; 273(40):25573-80.

Collino, Massimo, et al. "Modulation of the oxidative stress and inflammatory response by PPAR-γ agonists in the hippocampus of rats exposed to cerebral ischemia/reperfusion." European journal of pharmacology 530.1 (2006): 70-80.

Costa M, et al, "Investigation of endocannabinoid system genes suggests association between peroxisome proliferator activator receptor-alpha gene (PPARA) and schizophrenia." European Psychopharmacology, 2012.

Costa B, et al. "The non-psychoactive cannabis constituent cannabidiol is an orally effective therapeutic agent in rat chronic inflammatory and neuropathic pain." 2007.

Croxford and Yamamura. "Cannabinoids and the immune system: potential for the treatment of inflammatory diseases?" 2005.

d'Agostino G, et al. "Palmitoylethanolamide Protects Against the Amyloid-β25-35-Induced Learning and Memory Impairment in Mice, an Experimental Model of Alzheimer Disease." 2012.

De Oliveira AC, et al. "In vitro inhibition of CYP2B1 monooxygenase by beta-myrcene and other monoterpenoid compounds." 1997.

De Oliveira AC, Ribeiro-Pinto LF, Paumgartten JR. "In vitro inhibition of CYP2B1 monooxygenase by beta-myrcene and other monoterpenoid compounds." Toxicol Lett. 1997.

Di Marzo et al. "Bioactive long chain N-acylethanolamines in five species of edible bivalve molluscs." 1998.

DiMarzo et al. "Kavalactones and the endocannabinoid system: the plant-derived yangonin is a novel CB_1 receptor ligand." Pharmacological Research Journal. August 2012.

Dobrosi N, Toth BI, Nagy G, Dozsa A, Geczy T, Nagy G, et al. "Endocannabinoids enhance lipid synthesis and apoptosis of human sebocytes via cannabinoid receptor-2-mediated signaling." FASEB J. 2008

Duncan, M, Mouihate, A, Mackie, K., Keenan, CM, Buckley, NE, Davison, JS, Patel, KD, Pittman, QJ, Sharkey, KA. "Cannabinoid CB2 receptors in the enteric nervous system modulate gastrointestinal motility in Lipopolysaccharide-treated rats." Am J Physiol Gastrointest Liver Physiol 2008; 295: G78-G87.

E. Rozema, A. G. Atanasov, and B. Kopp. "Selected Extracts of Chinese Herbal Medicines: Their Effect on NF-κB, PPARα and PPARγ and the Respective Bioactive Compounds" 2012. Immunobiology, Volume 215, Issue 8, Pages 598-605.

ElSohly HN, Turner CE, Clark AM, ElSohly MA. "Effects of Linalool on glutamatergic system in the rat cerebral cortex." Neurochem Res. 1995

Esposito G, De Filippis D, Maiuri MC, De Stefano D, Carnuccio R, Iuvone T. "Cannabidiol inhibits inducible nitric oxide synthase protein expression and nitric oxide production in beta-amyloid stimulated PC12 neurons through p38 MAP kinase and NF-kappaB involvement." Neurosci Lett. 2006.

Esposito G, De Filippis D, Maiuri MC, De Stefano D, Carnuccio R, Luvone T. "Neurobiology: odorant receptors make scents." Nature. 2004; 430:511–512.

Esposito G, et al. "Cannabidiol inhibits inducible nitric oxide synthase protein expression and nitric oxide production in beta-amyloid stimulated PC12 neurons through p38 MAP kinase and NF-kappaB involvement." 2006.

Esposito G, et al. "Cannabidiol reduces amyloid beta-induced neuroinflammation and promotes hippocampal neurogenesis through PPAR-gamma involvement." PLOS One, 2011.

Esposito G, et al. "Neuroprotective effect of cannabidiol, a non-psychoactive component from Cannabis sativa, on beta-amyloid-induced toxicity in PC12 cells." 2004.

Falk-Filipsson A, et al. "Uptake, distribution and elimination of alpha-pinene in man after exposure by inhalation." 1990.

Falk-Filipsson A, Lof A, Hagberg M, Hjelm EW, Wang Z. "Uptake, distribution and elimination of alpha-pinene in man after exposure by inhalation. Scand J Work Environ Health." 1990

Fichna J., et al. "Endocannabinoid and cannabinoid-like fatty acid amide levels correlate with pain-related symptoms in patients with IBS-D and IBS-C: a pilot study." PLoS One 8:e85073, 2013.

Fischedick JT, et al. "D-limonene exposure to humans by inhalation: uptake, distribution, elimination, and effects on the pulmonary function." 1993.

Fischedick JT, et al. "Metabolic fingerprinting of Cannabis sativa L., cannabinoids and terpenoids for chemotaxonomic and drug standardization purposes." 2010.

Fischedick JT, Hazekamp A, Erkelens T, Choi YH, Verpoorte R. "d-limonene exposure to humans by inhalation: uptake, distribution, elimination, and effects on the pulmonary function." J Toxicol Environ Health. 1993
Fride E, Russo EB. Neuropsychiatry: Schizophrenia, depression, and anxiety. In: Onaivi E, Sugiura T, Di Marzo V, editors. "Metabolic fingerprinting of Cannabis sativa L., cannabinoids and terpenoids for chemotaxonomic and drug standardization purposes." Phytochem. 2010

Fukumoto S, et al. "Effect of flavour components in lemon essential oil on physical or psychological stress." 2008.

Fukumoto S, Morishita A, Furutachi K, Terashima T, Nakayama T, Yokogoshi H. "Effect of flavour components in lemon essential oil on physical or psychological stress." Stress Health. 2008;24:3–12.

Gerdeman GL, Lovinger DM. "Emerging roles for endocannabinoids in long-term synaptic plasticity." 2003.

Gerdeman GL, Lovinger DM. Gertsch J. "Emerging roles for endocannabinoids in long-term synaptic plasticity." Br J Pharmacol. 2003

Gertsch J, et al. "Anti-inflammatory cannabinoids in diet: towards a better understanding of CB(2) receptor action." 2008.

Gertsch J, Leonti M, Raduner S, Racz I, Chen JZ, Xie XQ, et al. "Anti-inflammatory cannabinoids in diet: towards a better understanding of CB(2) receptor action." Commun Integr Biol. 2008

Ghelardini C, Galeotti N, Salvatore G, Mazzanti G. "Beta-caryophyllene is a dietary cannabinoid." 2008.

Ghelardini C, Galeotti N, Salvatore G, Mazzanti G. "Beta-caryophyllene is a dietary cannabinoid." Proc Natl Acad Sci USA. 2008.

Gil ML, Jimenez J, Ocete MA, Zarzuelo A, Cabo MM. "Local anaesthetic activity of the essential oil of Lavandula angustifolia." Planta Med. 1999

Gorzalka BB. "Is there a role for the endocannabinoid system in the etiology and treatment of melancholic depression?" Behav Pharmacol. 2005. Hill MN,

Gomes-Carneiro MR, Viana ME, Felzenszwalb I, Paumgartten FJ. "Evaluation of beta-myrcene, alpha-terpinene and (+)- and (-)-alpha-pinene in the Salmonella/microsome assay." Food Chem Toxicol. 2005

Greenbaum L., et al. "Contribution of genetic variants to pain susceptibility in Parkinson disease." Eur J Pain 16:1243–1250., 2012.

Grotenhermen, Franjo. "Cannabinoids". Current Drug Target -CNS & Neurological Disorders. 2005.

Grotenhermen F, Russo EB, editors. Cannabis and Cannabinoids. "Non-cannabinoids in cannabis." In: Binghamton, NY: NY: Haworth Press; 2001.

Guzmán-Gutiérrez SL, et al. "Linalool and β-pinene exert their antidepressant-like activity through the monoaminergic pathway." Life Sci. 2015 May 1; 128:24-9. Epub 2015 Mar 11.

Hansen HS, Artmann, A. "Endocannabinoids and nutrition." J Neuroendocrinol. 2008 May;20 Suppl 1:94-9.

Hicks, John. "The Medicinal Power of Cannabis: Using a Natural Herb to Heal Arthritis, Nausea, Pain, and Other Ailments." 2015.

Hicks, John. "The Medicinal Power of Cannabis: Using a Natural Herb to Heal Arthritis, Nausea, Pain, and Other Ailments (p. 152)." Skyhorse Publishing. Kindle Edition. Other Ailments. 2015.

Hill MN., et al. "Serum endocannabinoid content is altered in females with depressive disorders: a preliminary report." Pharmacopsychiatry 41:48–53 2008.

Izzo AA, Borrelli F, Capasso R, Di Marzo V, Mechoulam R. "Non-psychotropic plant cannabinoids: new therapeutic opportunities from an ancient herb." Trends Pharmacol Sci. 2009

Jocelijn Meijerink, Michiel Balvers, and Renger Witkamp. "N-acyl amines of docosahexaenoic acid and other n–3 polyunsatured fatty acids – from fishy endocannabinoids to potential leads." Br J Pharmacol. 2013 Jun; 169(4): 772–783.

John M. McPartland. "The Endocannabinoid System, An Osteopathic Perspective." The Journal of the American Osteopathic Association, October 2008, Vol. 108, 586-600. DO October 2008

Jonsson KO1, Vandevoorde S, Lambert DM, Tiger G, Fowler CJ. "Effects of homologues and analogues of palmitoylethanolamide upon the inactivation of the endocannabinoid anandamide. Br J Pharmacol. 2001 Aug; 133(8):1263-75.

Jürg Gertsch, Roger G Pertwee, and Vincenzo Di Marzo. "Phytocannabinoids beyond the Cannabis plant – do they exist?" British Journal of Pharmacology, 2010, 160: 523–529.

Katsuyama S., Mizoguchi H., Kuwahata H.; et al. "Involvement of peripheral cannabinoid and opioid receptors in β-caryophyllene-induced antinociception." (2013). European journal of pain 17 (5): 664–675.

Kaufmann I., Hauer D., Huge V., et al. "Enhanced anandamide plasma levels in patients with complex regional pain syndrome following traumatic injury: a preliminary report." Eur Surg Res 43:325–329. 2009.

Kent D. Chapman, Barney Venables, Chris Bettinger et al. "N-Acylethanolamines in Seeds. Quantification of Molecular Species and Their Degradation upon Imbibition." 1999.

Kim SS, Baik JS, Oh TH, Yoon WJ, Lee NH, Hyun CG. "Treatment with lavender aromatherapy in the post-anesthesia care unit reduces opioid requirements of morbidly obese patients undergoing laparoscopic adjustable gastric banding." Obes Surg. 2007

King AR, Dotsey EY, Lodola A, Jung KM, Ghomian A, Qiu Y, et al. "Discovery of potent and reversible monoacylglycerol lipase inhibitors." Chem Biol. 2009; 16:1045–1052.

Koethe D., et al. "Expression of CB1 cannabinoid receptor in the anterior cingulate cortex in schizophrenia, bipolar disorder, and major depression." J Neural Transm 114:1055–1063. 2007.

Komiya, M, et al. "Lemon oil vapor causes an anti-stress effect via modulating the 5-HT and DA activities in mice." Behavior Brain Research 2006. 172 (2): 240-9.

Komori T, Fujiwara R, Tanida M, Nomura J, Yokoyama MM. "Effects of citrus fragrance on immune function and depressive states." Neuroimmunomodulation. 1995

Lambert DM, Di Marzo V. The palmitoylethanolamide and oleamide enigmas: are these two fatty acid amides cannabimimetic. Curr Med Chem. 1999; 6:757–773.

Lapczynski A, Bhatia SP, Letizia CS, Api AM. "Fragrance material review on nerolidol (isomer unspecified)" Food Chem Toxicol. 2008

Limei Wang, et al. "Natural product agonists of peroxisome proliferator-activated receptor gamma" (PPARγ): a review Biochem Pharmacol. 2014 Nov 1; 92(1): 73–89.

Lorenzetti BB, Souza GE, Sarti SJ, Santos Filho D, Ferreira SH. "Myrcene mimics the peripheral analgesic activity of lemongrass tea." J Ethnopharmacol. 1991

Lo Verme J, Fu J, Astarita G, La Rana G, Russo R, Calignano A, Piomelli D: The nuclear receptor peroxisome proliferator-activated receptor-alpha mediates the anti-inflammatory actions of palmitoylethanolamide. Mol Pharmacol 2005,67(1):15–19.

Iuvone T, Esposito G, Esposito R, Santamaria R, Di Rosa M, Izzo AA. "Neuroprotective effect of cannabidiol, a non-psychoactive component from Cannabis sativa, on beta-amyloid-induced toxicity in PC12 cells." J Neurochem. 2004; 89:134–141.

Mackie K. (2005) Distribution of cannabinoid receptors in the central and peripheral nervous system. Handb Exp Pharmacol 168:299–325.

Marzo, Vincenzo Di. "Cannabinoids (Neuroscience Intelligence Unit)" (1st ed.) (2004). Georgetown, Texas: Springer. pp. 99, 181.

Maurelli S, Bisogno T, De Petrocellis L, Di Luccia A, Marino G, Di Marzo V FEBS Lett. "Two novel classes of neuroactive fatty acid amides are substrates for mouse neuroblastoma 'anandamide amidohydrolase'." 1995 Dec 11; 377(1):82-6.

Mazzola, Carmen, et al. "Fatty acid amide hydrolase (FAAH) inhibition enhances memory acquisition through activation of PPAR-α nuclear receptors." Learning & Memory 16.5 (2009): 332-337.

McPartland JM, Russo EB. "Cannabis and cannabis extracts: greater than the sum of their parts?" J Cannabis Therap. 2001.

McPartland JM, Pruitt PL. Side effects of pharmaceuticals not elicited by comparable herbal medicines: the case of tetrahydrocannabinol and marijuana. Altern Ther Health Med. 1999; 5:57–62.

Michael K. Racke, et al. "Nuclear Receptors and Autoimmune Disease: The Potential of PPAR Agonists to Treat Multiple Sclerosis" J. Nutr. Mar; 136(3)2006.

Mitjans M., et al. "Screening genetic variability at the CNR1 gene in both major depression etiology and clinical response to citalopram treatment." Psychopharmacology (Berl) 227:509–519. 2013.

Prakash Nagarkatti, Rupal Pandey, Mitzi Nagar et al. "Cannabinoids as novel anti-inflammatory drugs." Future Med Chemistry. Oct. 2009.

Reggio, Patricia. "Endocannabinoid Binding to the Cannabinoid Receptors: What Is Known and What Remains Unknown." Curr Med Chem. 2014 Aug 4.

Russo EB. "Clinical endocannabinoid deficiency (CECD): can this concept explain therapeutic benefits of cannabis in migraine, fibromyalgia, irritable bowel syndrome and other treatment-resistant conditions?" (2004) Neuro Endocrinol Lett 25: 31–39

Russo EB. "Taming THC: potential cannabis synergy and phytocannabinoid-terpenoid entourage effects." Br J Pharmacol. 2011 Aug; 163(7): 1344–1364.

Saravanan Kanakasabai, et al. "Peroxisome proliferator-activated receptor δ agonists inhibit T helper type 1 (Th1) and Th17 responses in experimental allergic encephalomyelitis." Immunology. 2010 Aug; 130(4): 572–588.

S.J., Diemel, L.T., Pryce, G., Baker, D. "The Medicinal Power of Cannabis: Using a Natural Herb to Heal Arthritis, Nausea, Pain, and Jackson Cannabinoids and neuroprotection in CNS inflammatory diseas." J. Neurol. Sci. 2005; 233: 21– 25.

Sadiye Amcaoglu Rieder, Ashok Chauhan, Ugra Singh, Mitzi Nagarkatti, Prakash Nagarkatti. "Cannabinoid-induced apoptosis in immune cells as a pathway to immunosuppression" 2010.

Salminen A, et al. "Terpenoids: natural inhibitors of NF-kappaB signaling with anti-inflammatory and anticancer potential." JCell Mol Life Sci. 2008 Oct;65(19):2979-99.

Sepe, Nunzio; De Petrocellis, Luciano; Montanaro, Francesca; Cimino, Guido; Di Marzo, Vincenzo. "Bioactive long chain N-acylethanolamines in five species of edible bivalve molluscs." (1998). Biochimica et Biophysica Acta (BBA) - Lipids and Lipid Metabolism 1389 (2): 101–11.

Smart D, Jonsson KO, Vandevoorde S, Lambert DM, Fowler CJ. "Entourage' effects of n-acyl ethanolamines at human vanilloid receptors. Comparison of effects upon anandamide-induced vanilloid receptor activation and upon anandamide metabolism." Br J Pharmacol. 2002

Spinella M. "The importance of pharmacological synergy in psychoactive herbal medicines." Altern Med Rev. April 2002.

Taylor & Francis. "Endocannabinoids: The Brain and Body's Marijuana and beyond." Boca Raton, FL: 2006.

Willson TM et al. "The PPARs: from orphan receptors to drug discovery." J Med Chem. 2000 Feb 24; 43 (4):527-50.

Wright K., et al. "Differential expression of cannabinoid receptors in the human colon: cannabinoids promote epithelial wound healing. Gastroenterology." 2005 Aug; 129(2):437-53.

Yu, Xin, et al. "Activation of cerebral peroxisome proliferator-activated receptors gamma exerts neuroprotection by inhibiting oxidative stress following pilocarpine-induced status epilepticus." Brain research 1200 (2008): 146-158.

"Aromatherapy: evidence for sedative effects of the essential oil of lavender after inhalation." Zaturforsch [C] 1991.

"The non-psychoactive cannabis constituent cannabidiol is an orally effective therapeutic agent in rat chronic inflammatory and neuropathic pain." Eur J Pharmacol. 2007.

"Aromatherapy: evidence for sedative effects of the essential oil of lavender after inhalation." Z Naturforsch [C] 1991